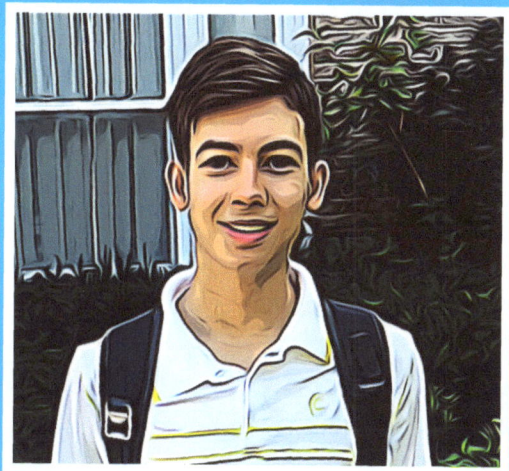

About The Author

Elliot Bloom is a Sophomore from the Northwest suburbs of Chicago. He has dealt with a life-threatening nut allergy since he was three. This heavily restricted his food options, but made him very attentive at reading the ingredients in any packaged food.

This book is based on Elliot's childhood incident. He wrote it in order to spread awareness about the dangers of food allergies, specifically in school environments.

ISBN: 979-8-218-09358-7

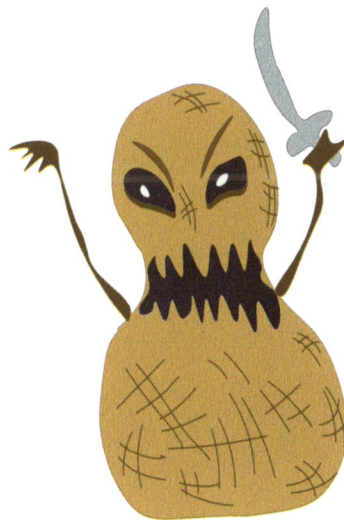

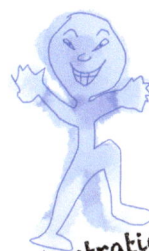

Illustrations by:
Eno Bloom

1

A Boy Called Peanut

Once upon a time, there was a little boy named Elliot.
Elliot was small, cute, funny and curious.

His Mama called him Peanut.

He was a perfectly healthy and happy little boy, who liked cars, trucks, airplanes and soccer.

AKA: Elliot

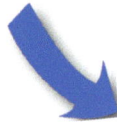

Favorite food?

His favorite food was macaroni and cheese.
In fact, he loved it so much that he would eat all his broccoli first, as long as it was followed by macaroni & cheese.

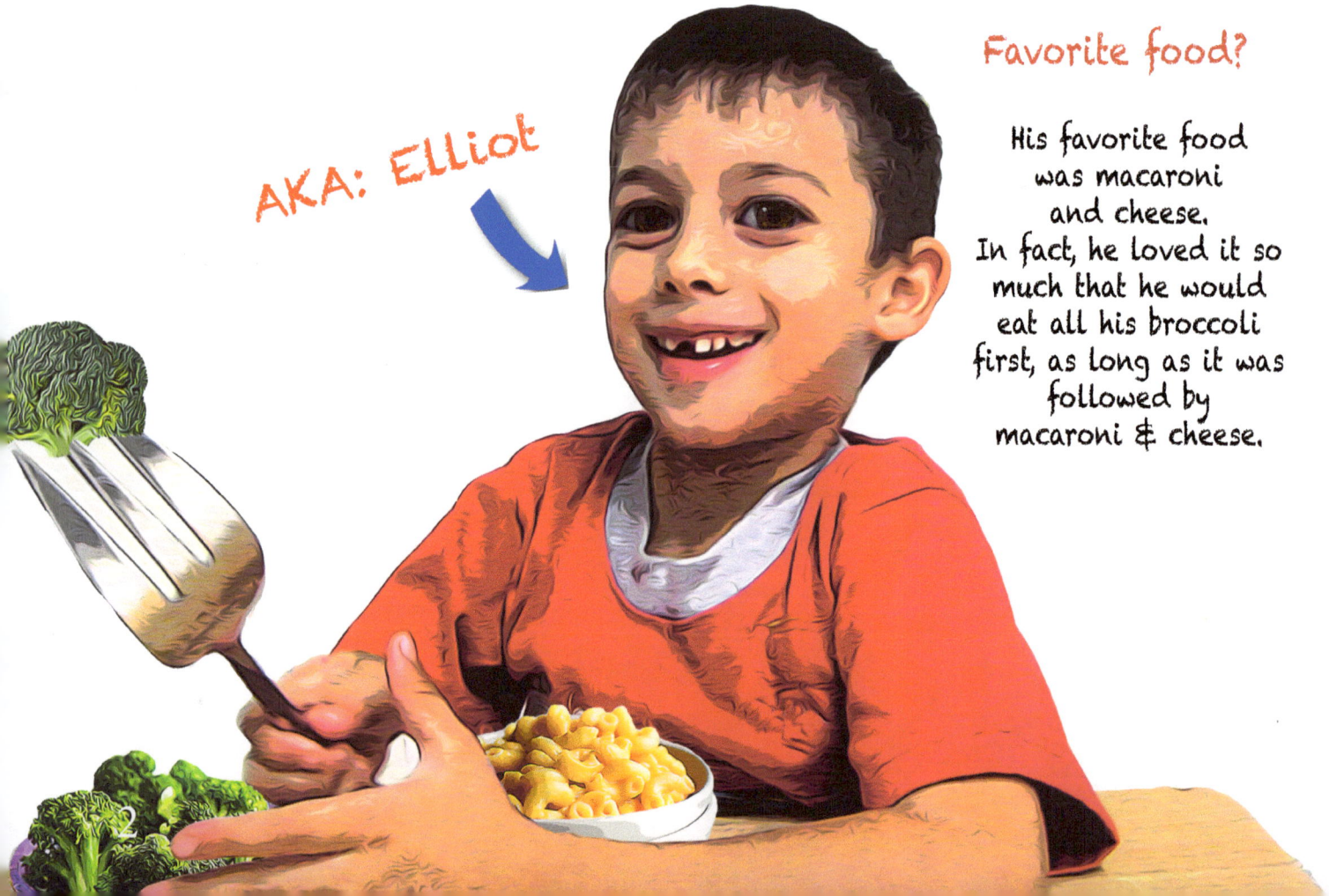

Big Outing

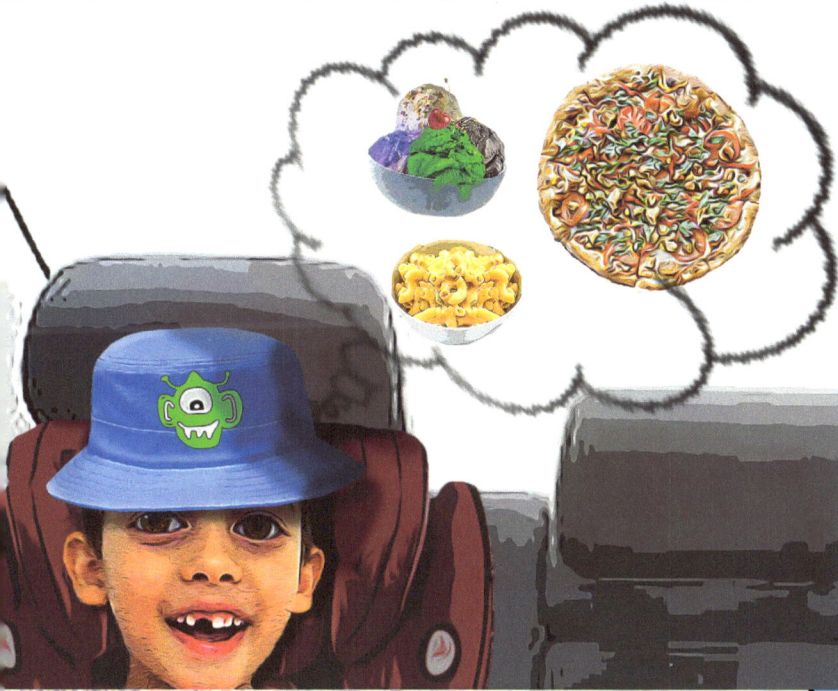

One day, Mama, Papa, big brother Isaac, and Elliot went to a new restaurant. Elliot loved visiting new places, seeing all the new types of food and meeting new people.

During the whole car ride to the restaurant, Elliot could not stop thinking about all the food he was going to enjoy.

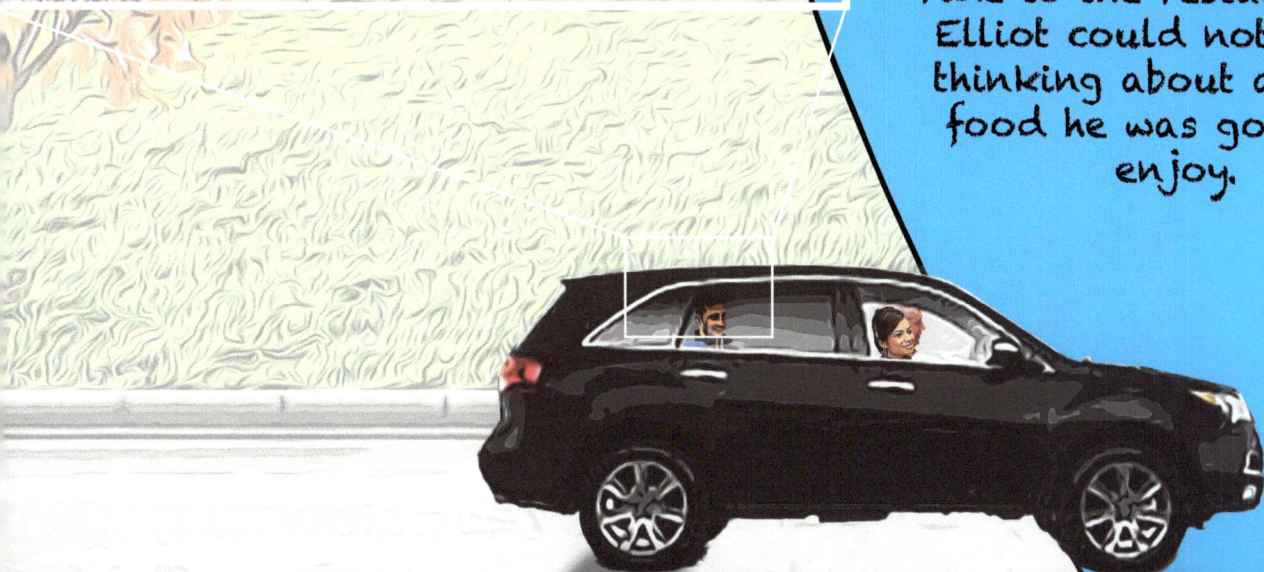

Hungry Boy!

Mama ordered a salad, so that Elliot could eat his vegetables. She was all about the veggies! The whole family laughed when they saw the name of the salad, "Peanut Salad, family size."

"Hey, that salad must be for me!" Elliot said.

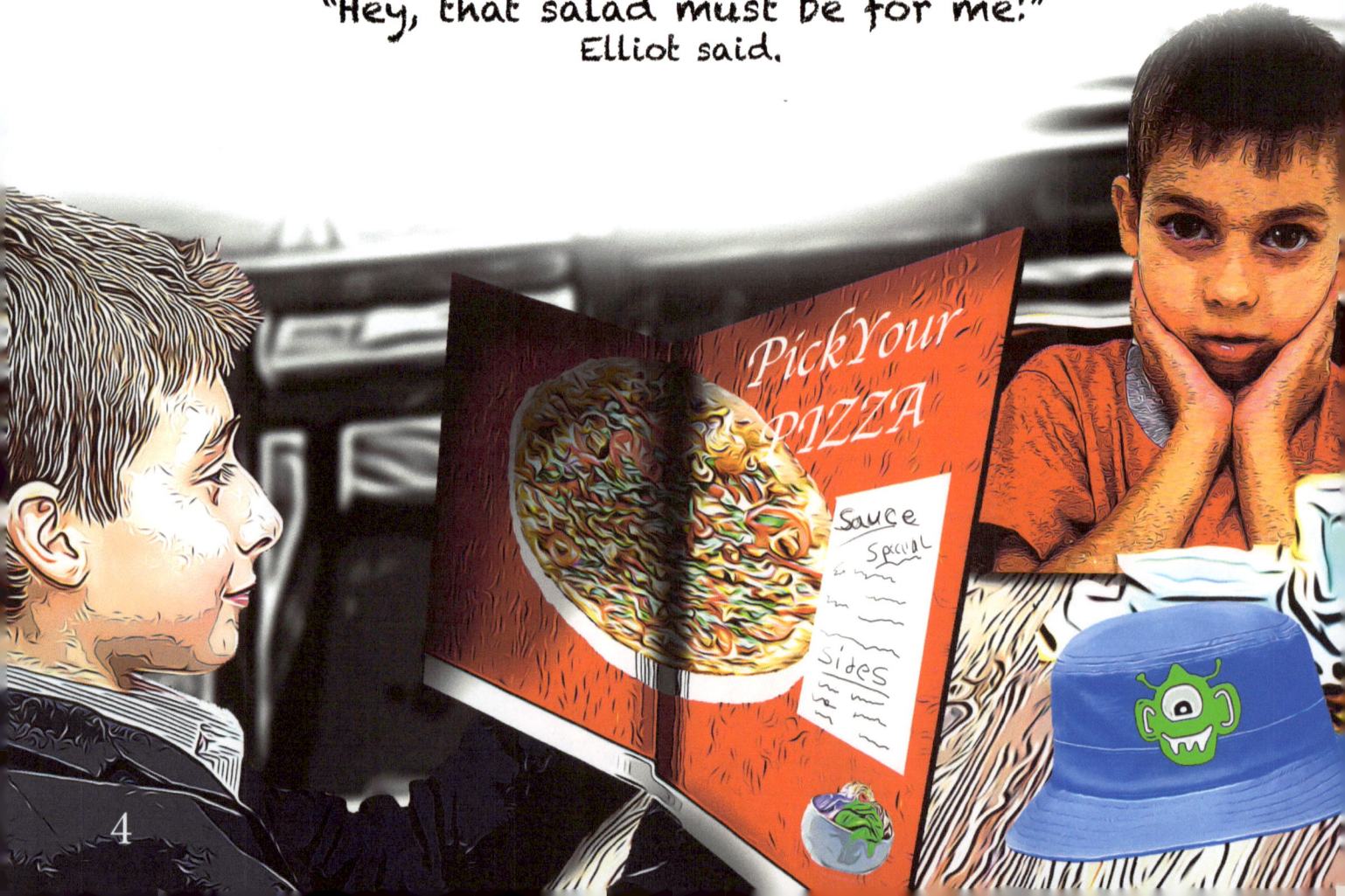

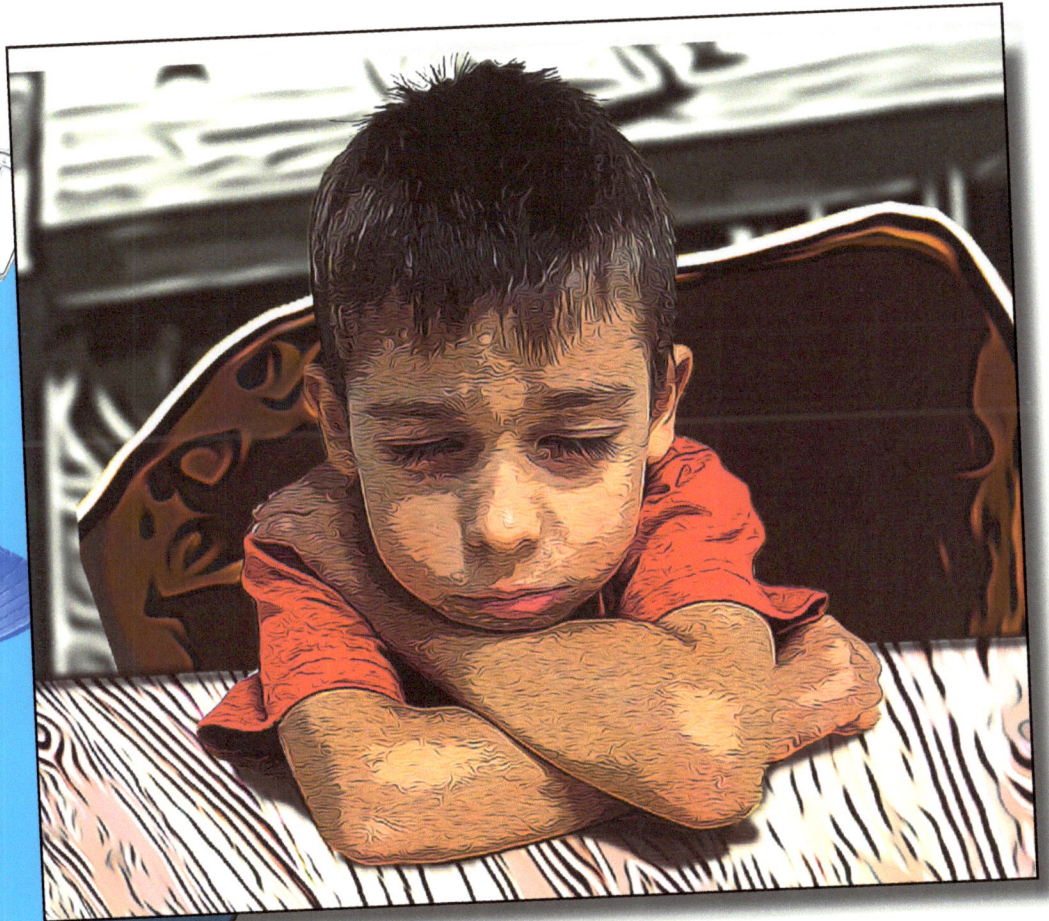

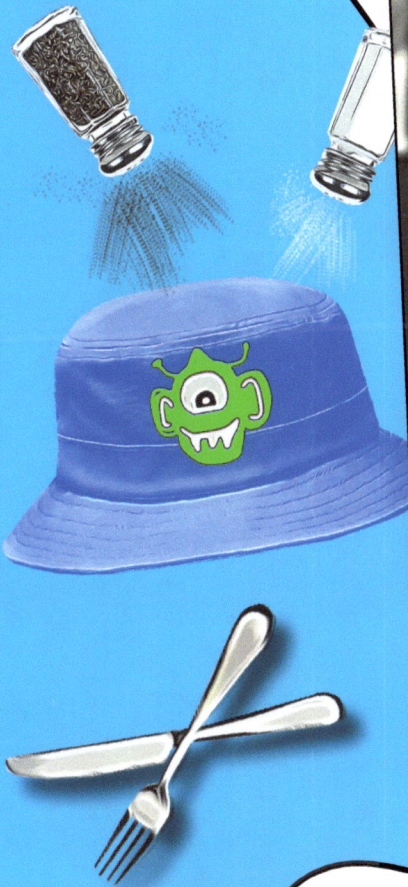

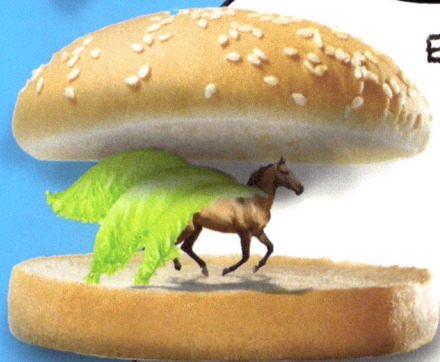

Elliot was very hungry and he closed his eyes and said –

"I'm hungry, I want to eat a horse!
I'm so hungry I could eat my hat!"

Time to Eat!

The waiter brought the salad.
"I bet I know who is going to get the first bite!"
said the waiter.

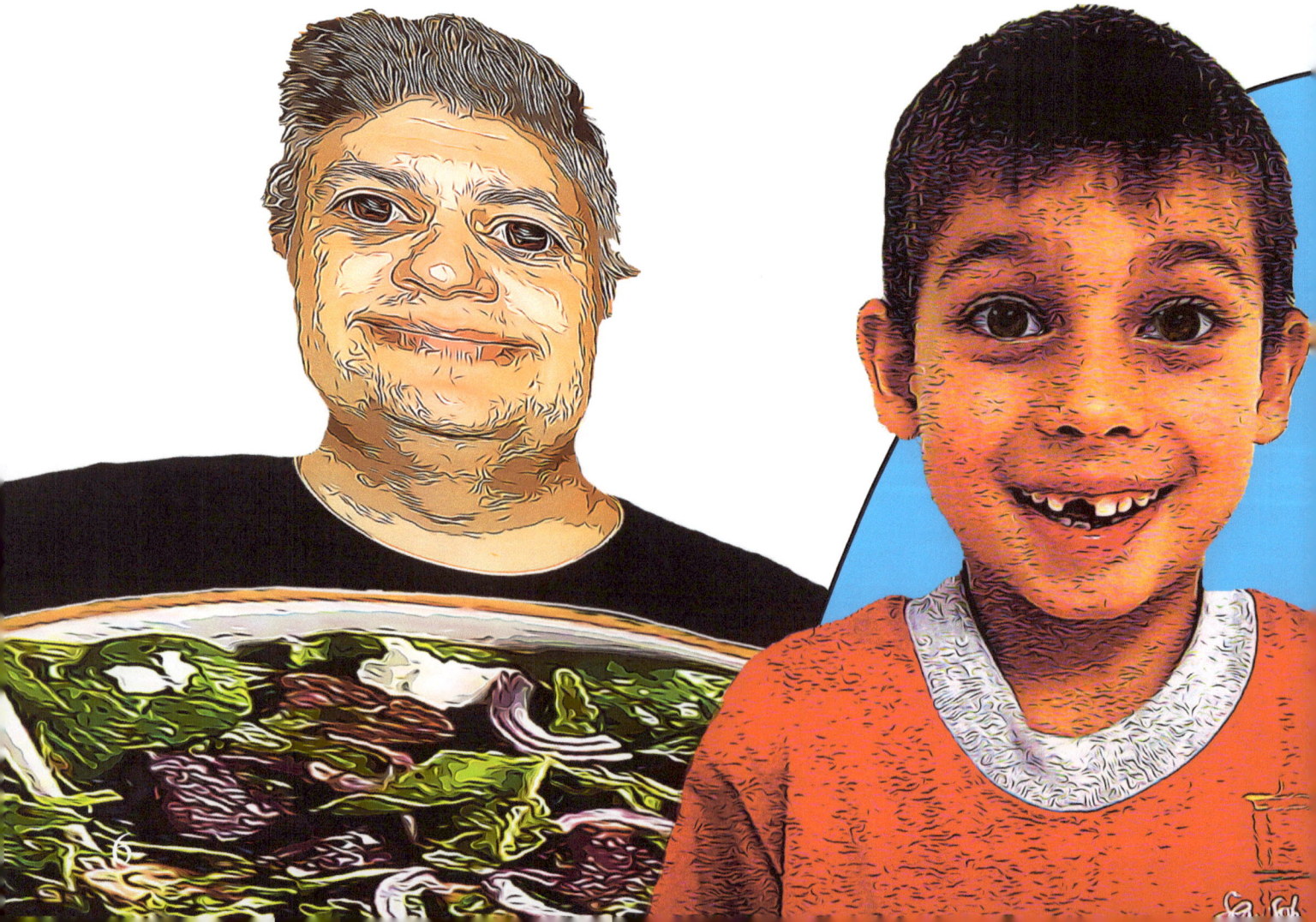

Elliot started to eat .....

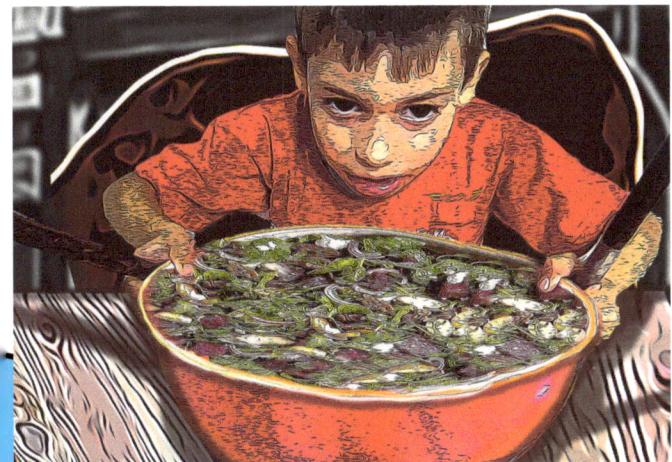

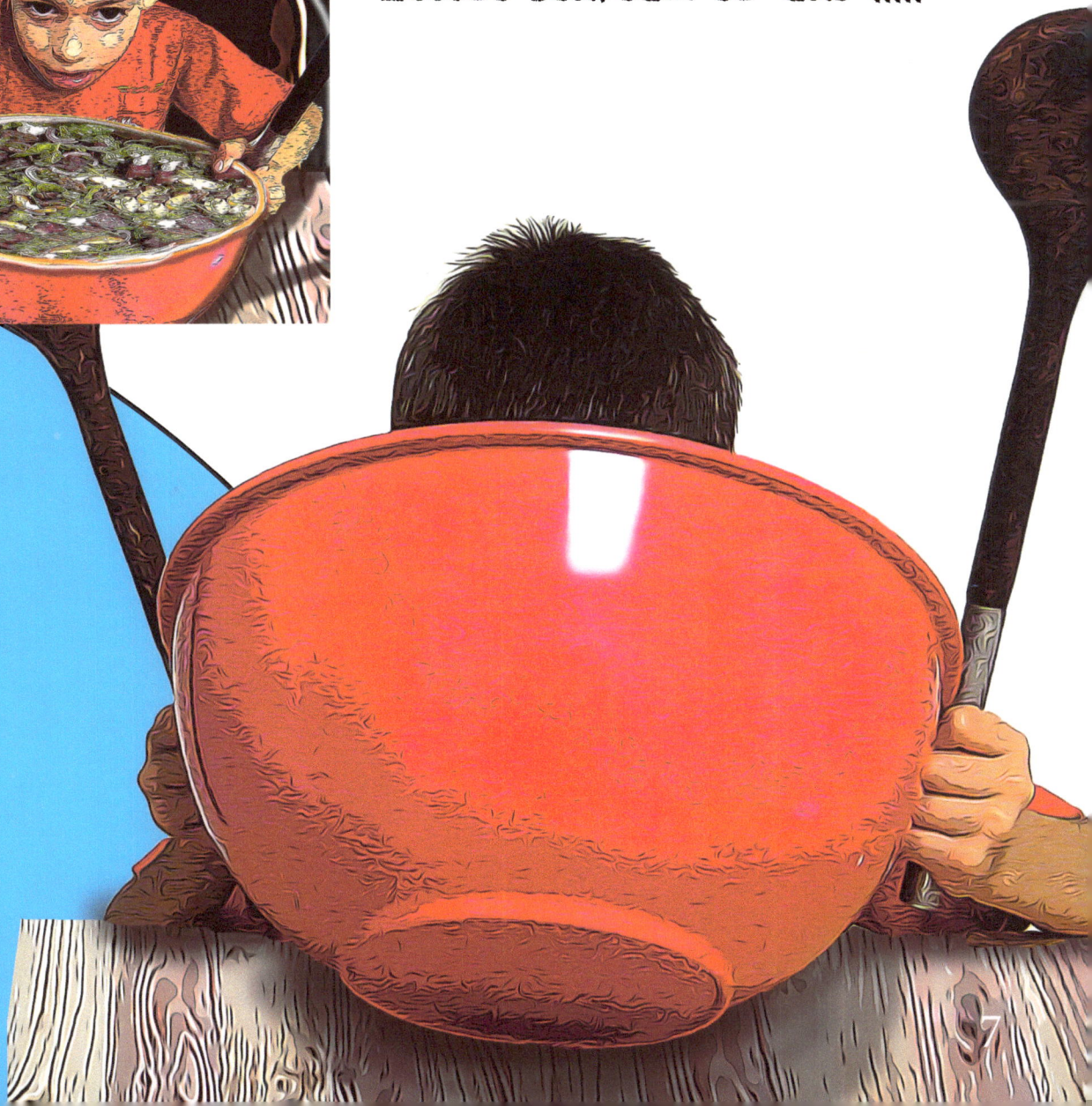

Something Happened

He was
very happy!

Elliot started to rub his eyes.
"What is wrong baby?"

Mama noticed that the area
around his eyes became red.

Elliot started to get
uncomfortable.

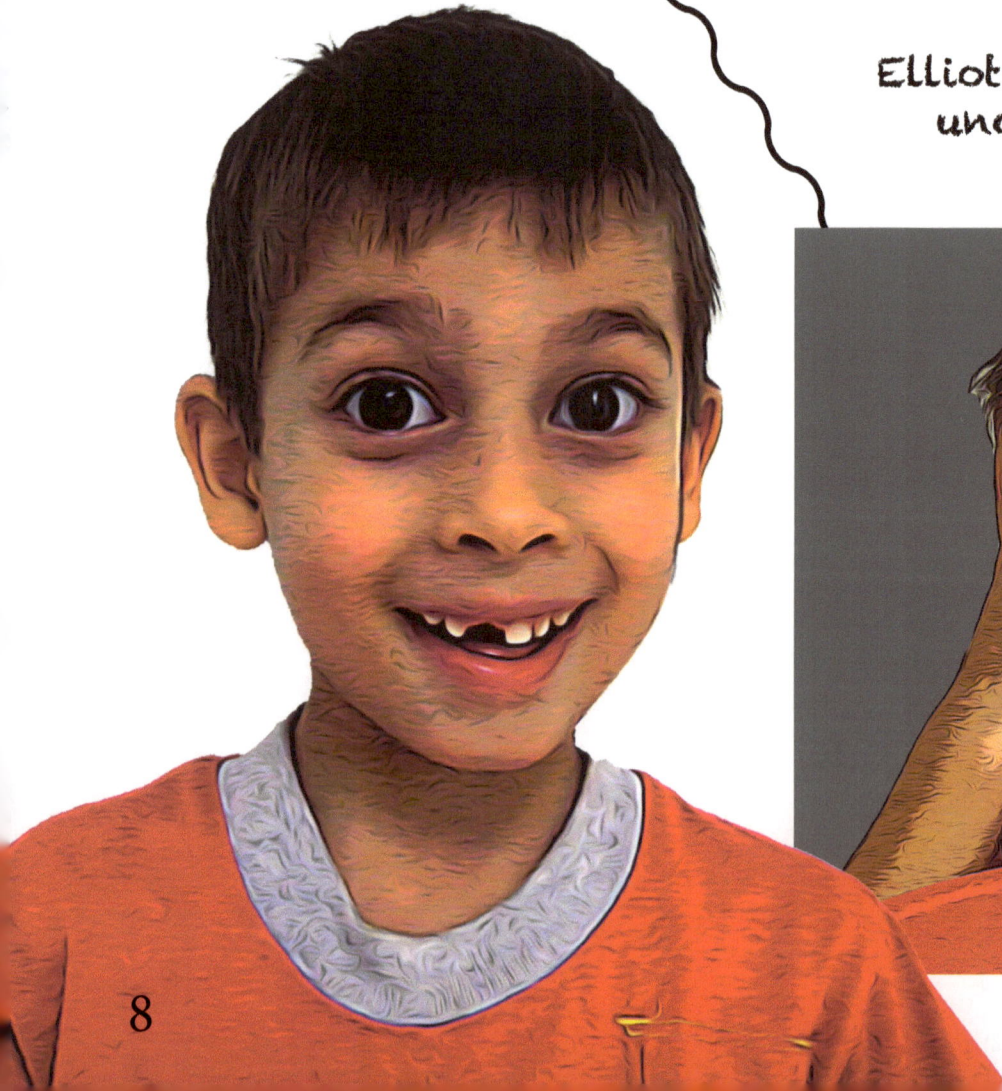

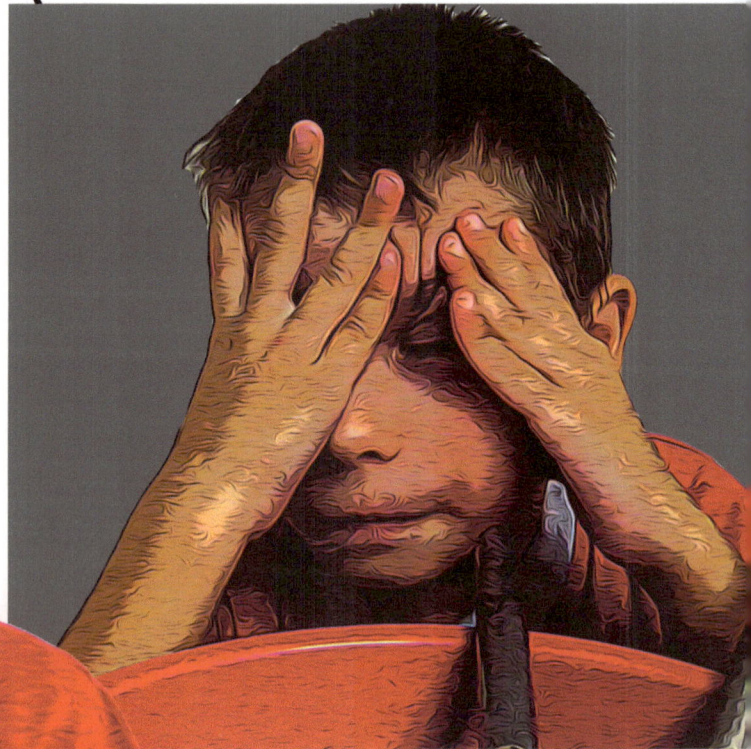

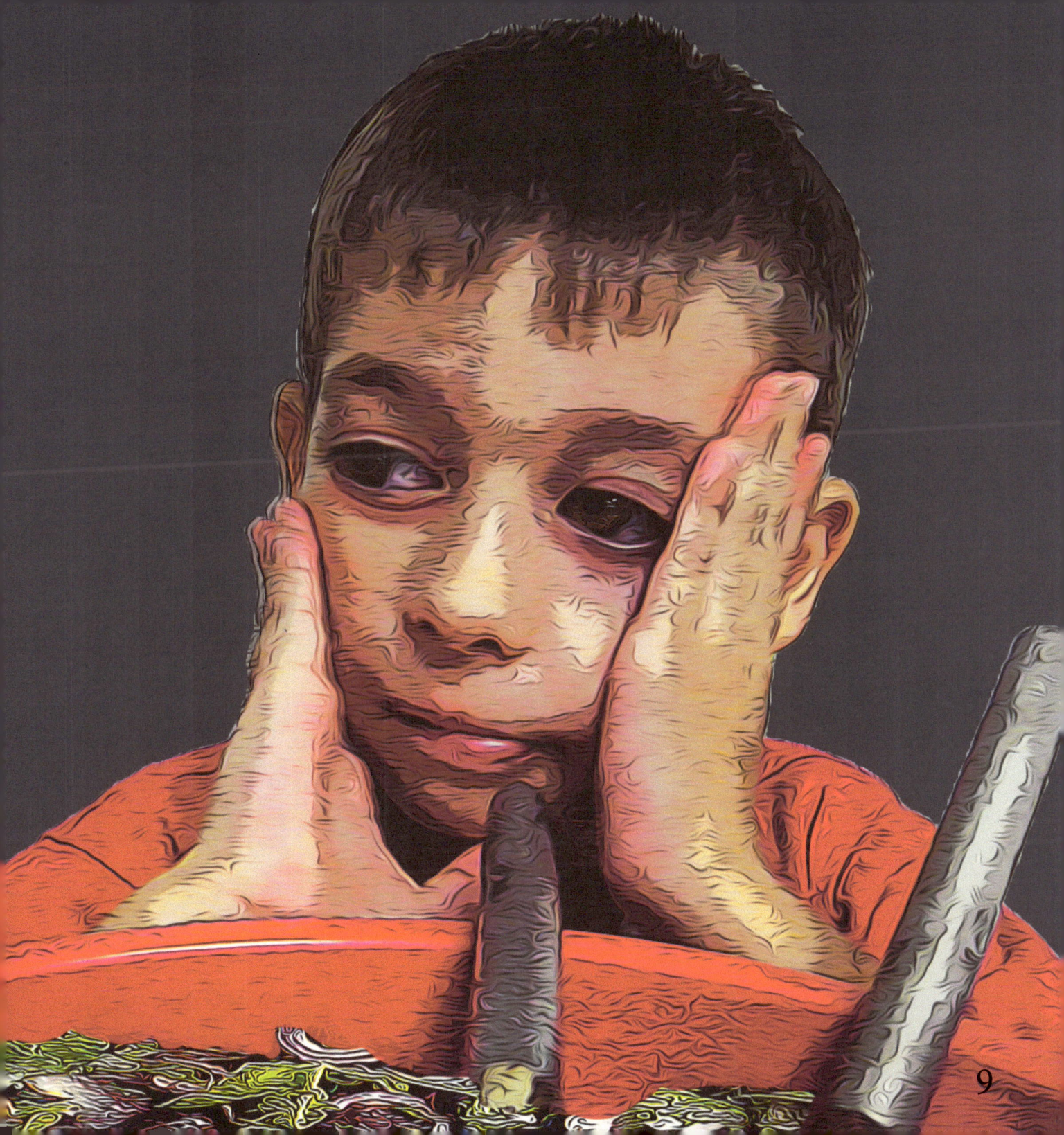

Papa remembered a friend that had an allergy and would react this way when he ate something he was not supposed to eat.

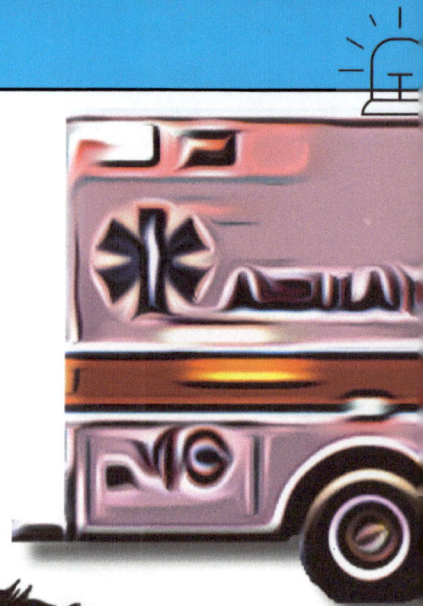

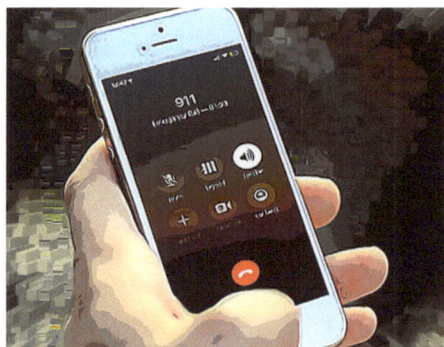

Papa dialed 911

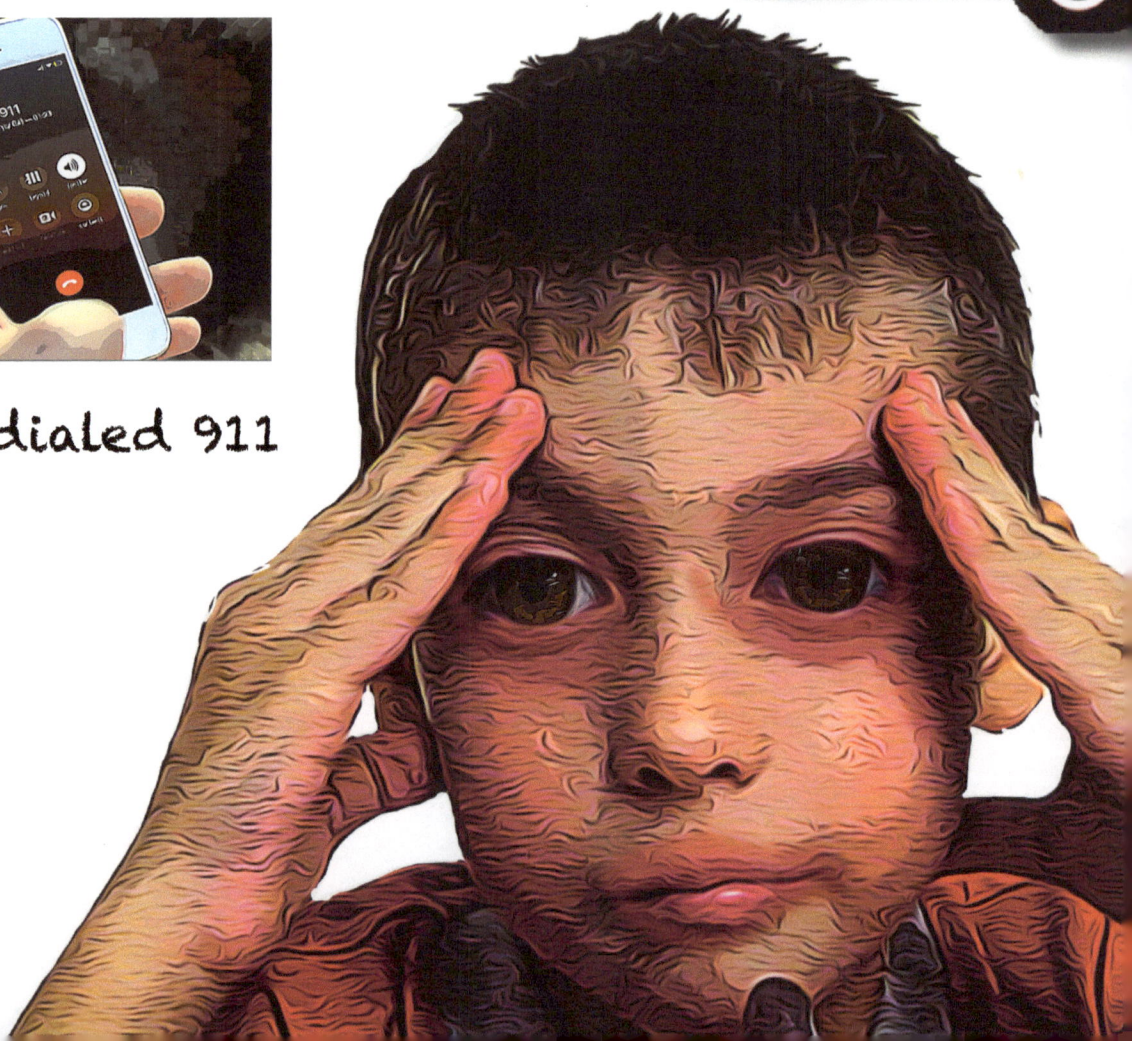

A Close Encounter

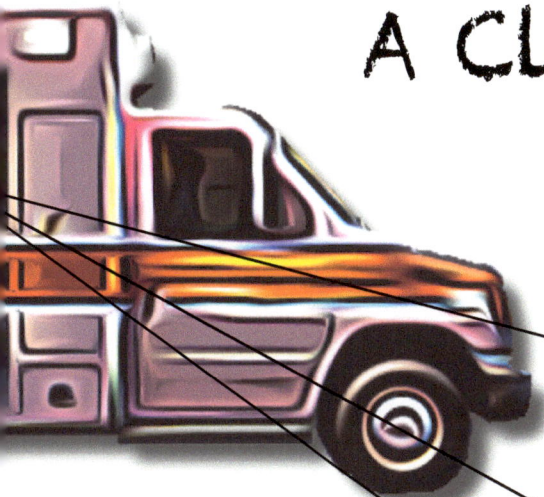

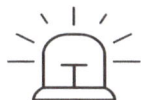

Elliot always loved to see ambulances and fire trucks, but at this moment, he was not feeling so well.

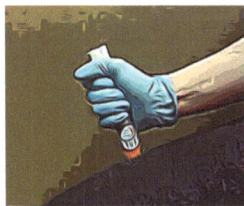

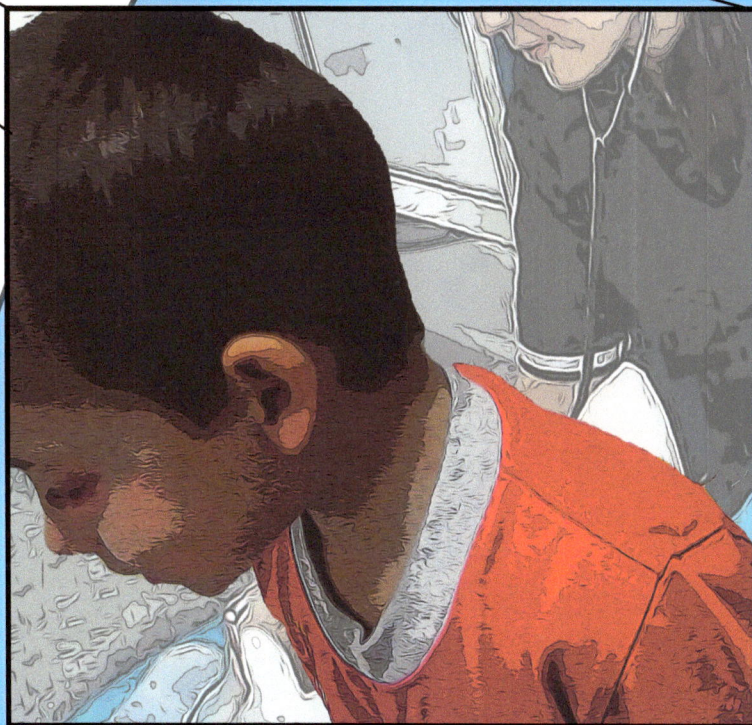

Lucky Boy

The doctors asked Mama and Papa many questions at the hospital.

Elliot remembered everything that was going on in the ambulance after they pinched his leg.

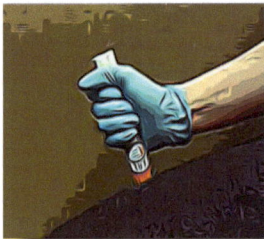

It was a strange pinching tool.

Elliot thought, 'Maybe, unlike my brother's pinches, a doctor's pinch is healing.'

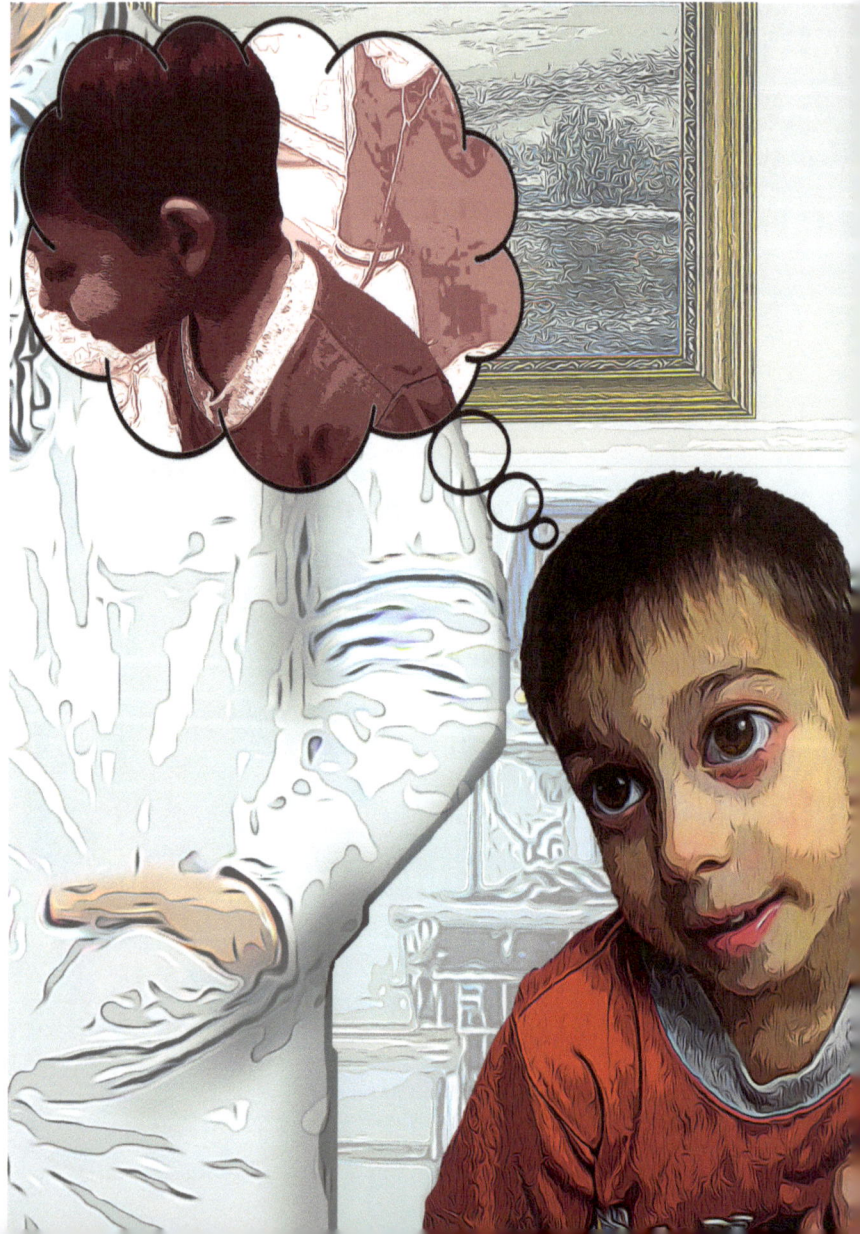

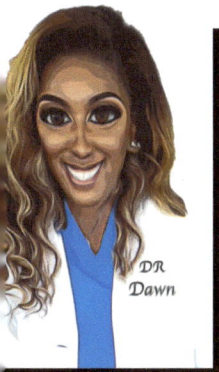

The doctor told Elliot that he had an allergy to nuts, specifically peanuts and a few other nuts.

"It means that you cannot have certain foods because your body thinks they are trying to hurt you."

"Do you know what made Superman lose his superpowers?" asked the doctor.

"Yes," said Elliot, "it was kryptonite...."

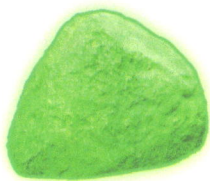

"That's right Elliot. Superman was allergic to kryptonite. So, you are very similar to Superman, but your kryptonite happens to be nuts."

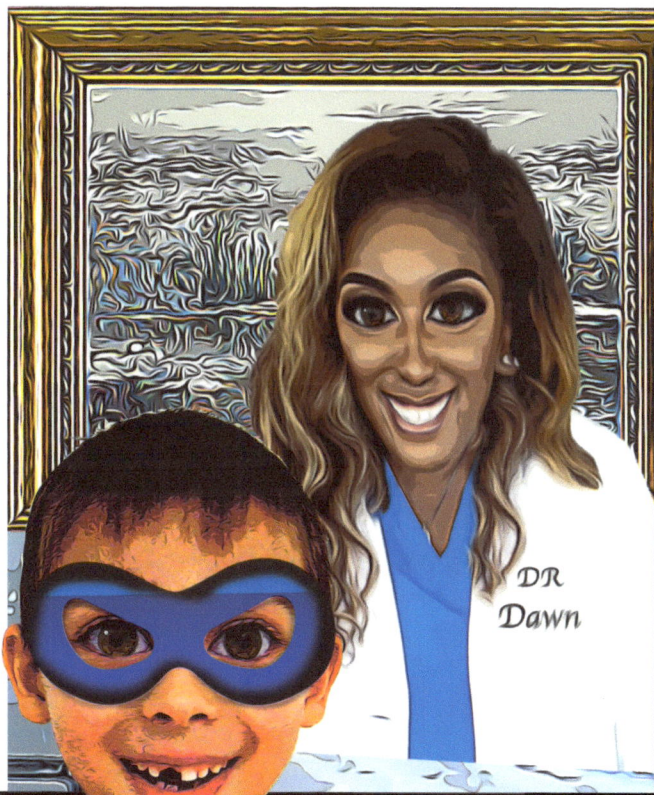

Super Boy!!

Elliot was quiet for a moment and asked the doctor if he has superpowers like Superman.

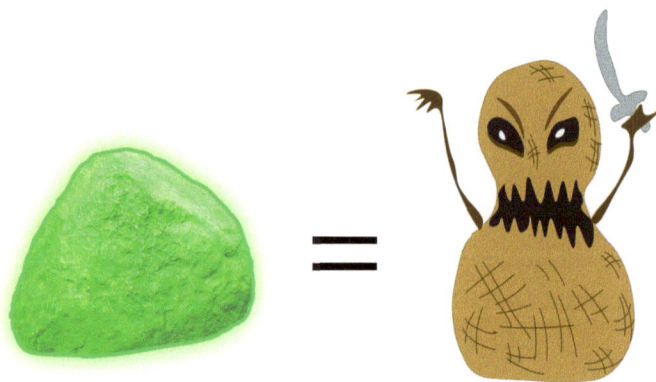

The doctor smiled and told Elliot that he's a super kid and has allergies just like Superman.

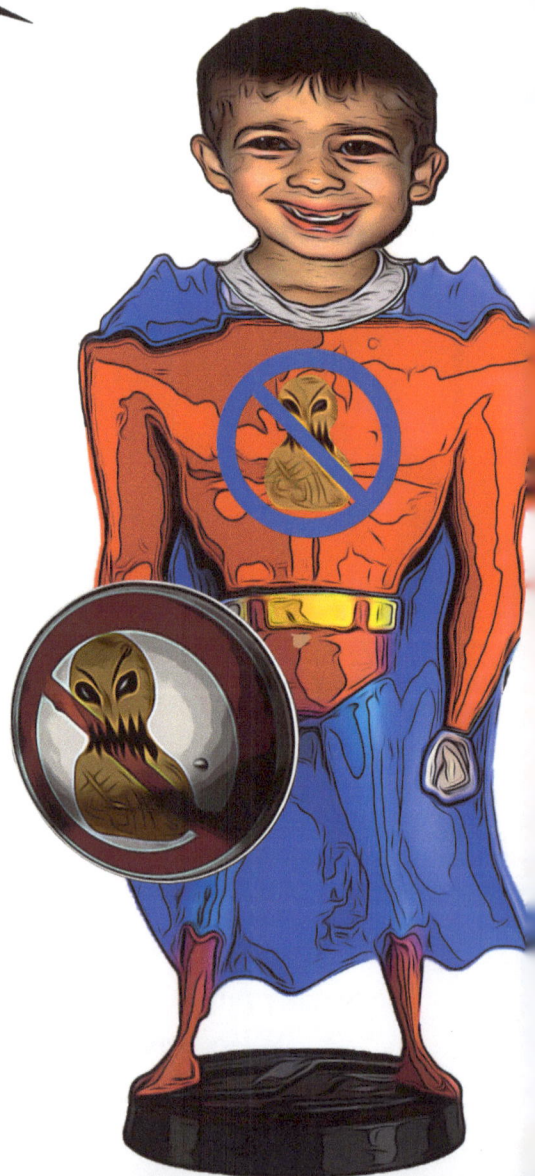

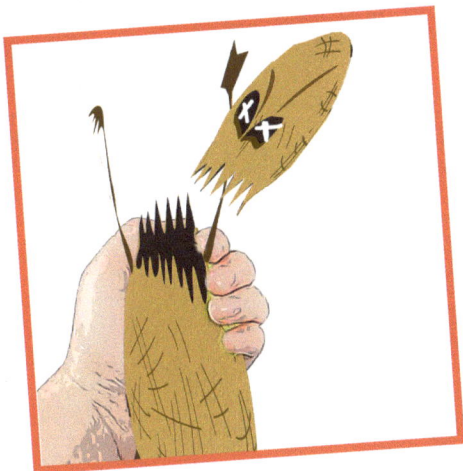

"Now, we have to help you protect yourself from the things that you are allergic to."

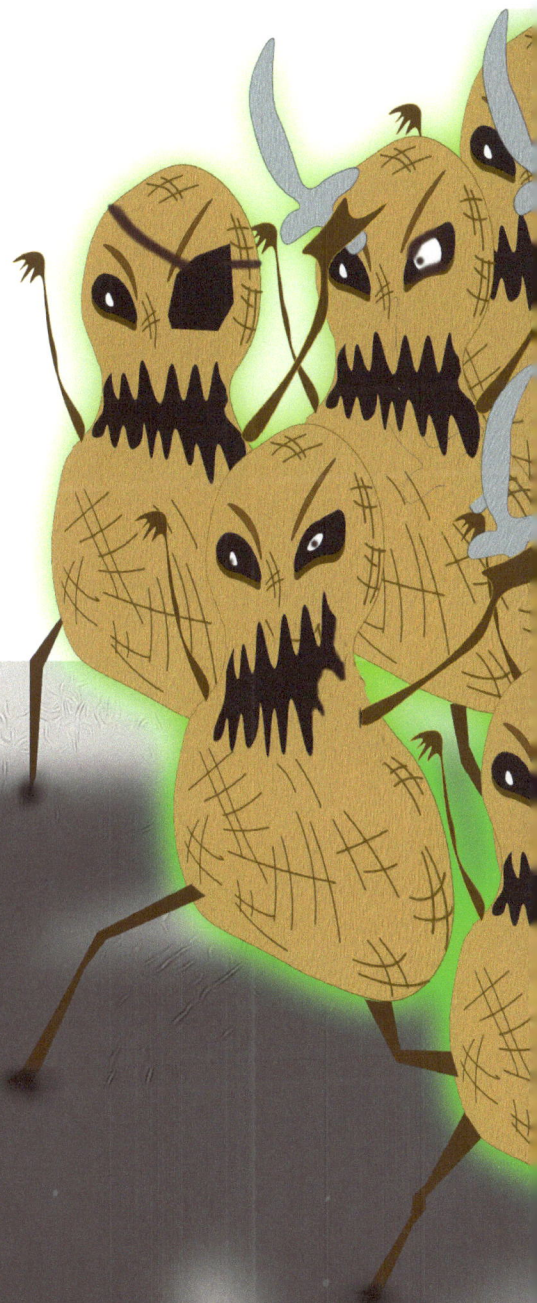

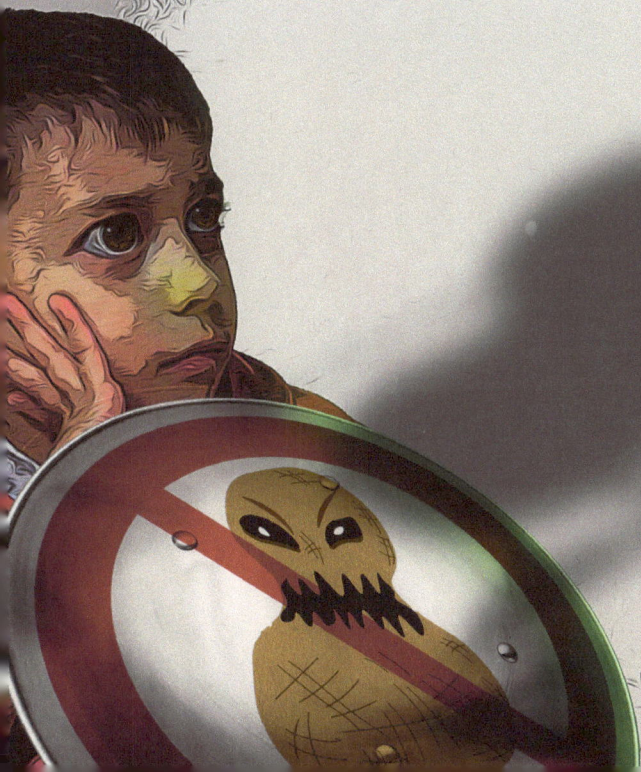

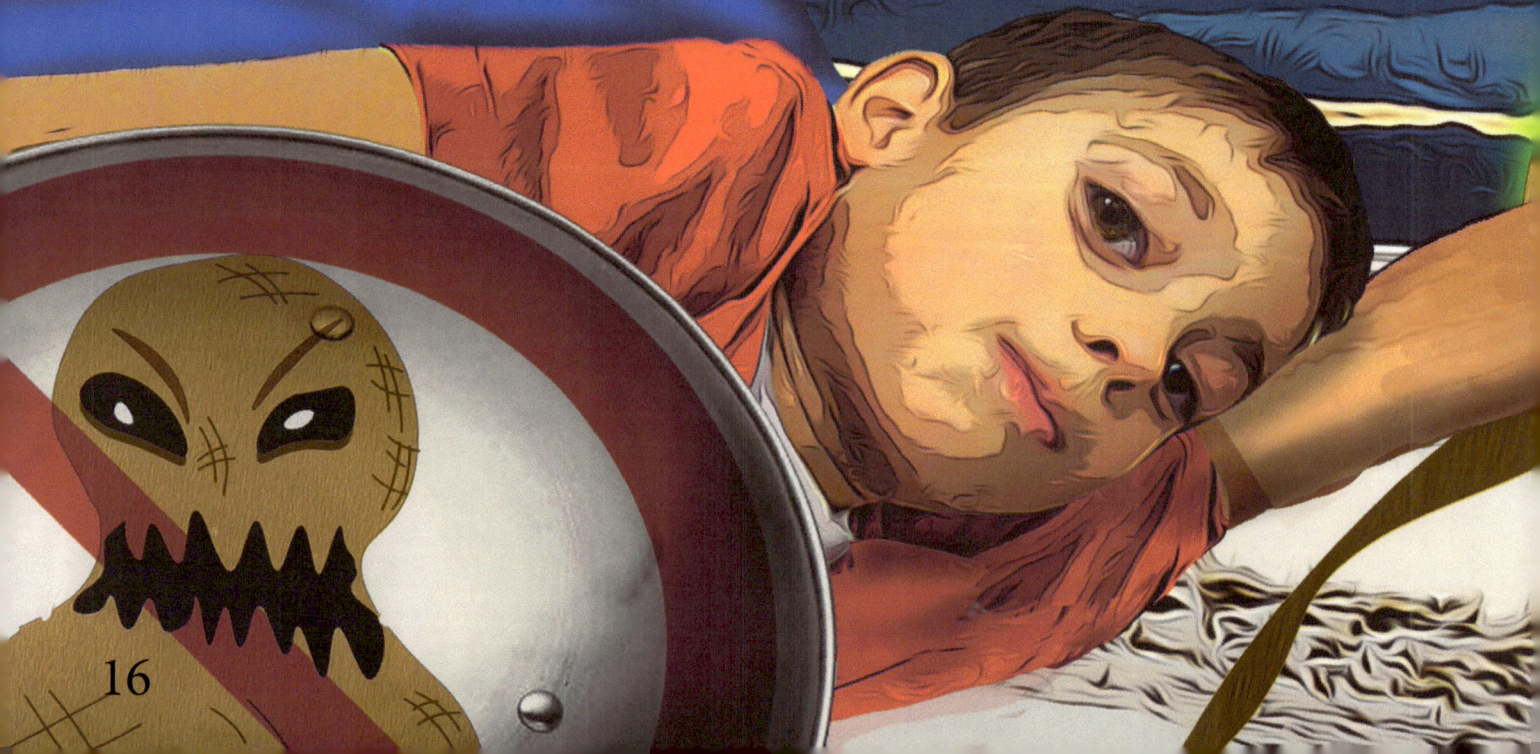

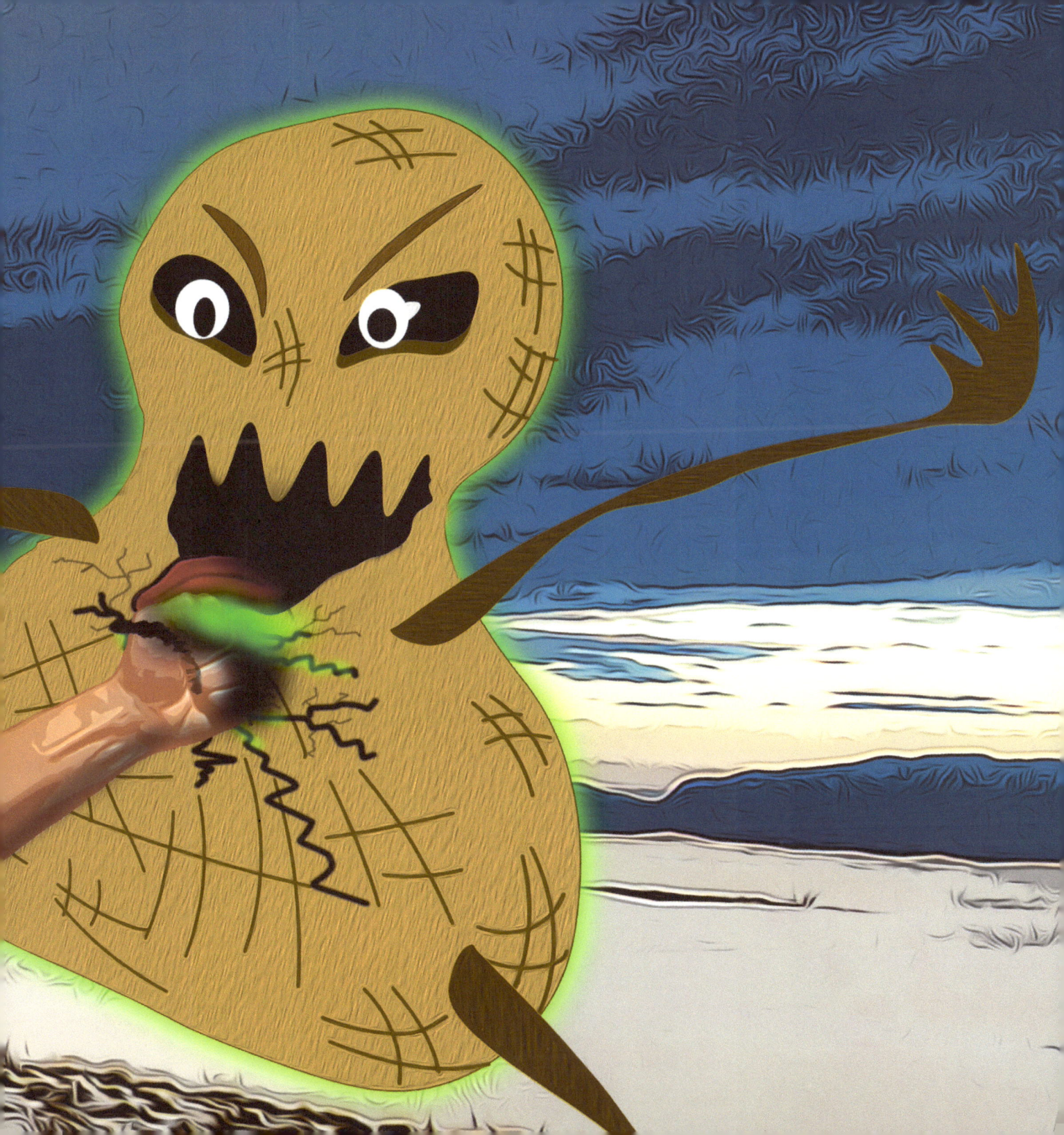

Education

You and your family will have to be very careful with what you eat, where you go to eat, and where the food is made. You need to always ask an adult before you eat something, and you need to educate the people around you about what an allergy is and how dangerous it can be.

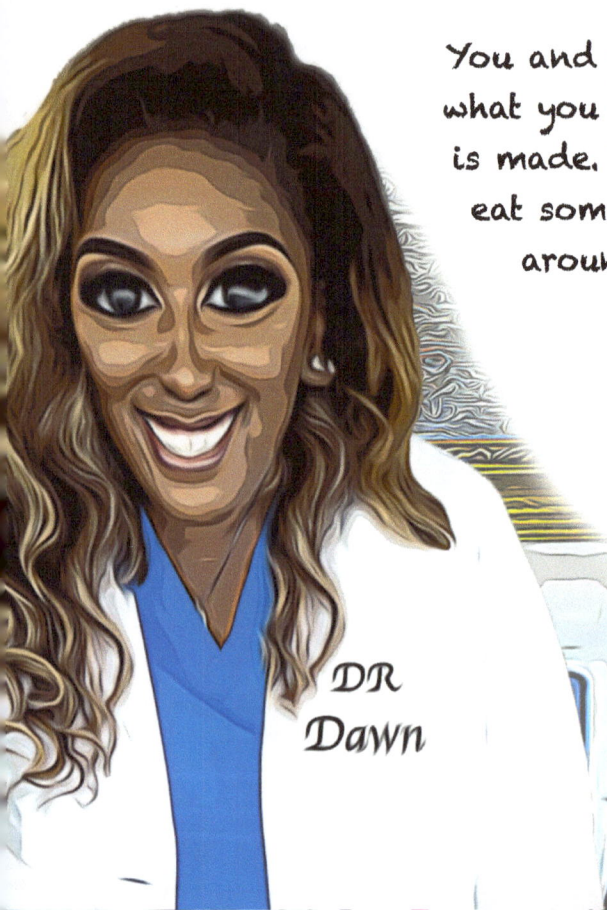

DR Dawn

NO PEANUTS

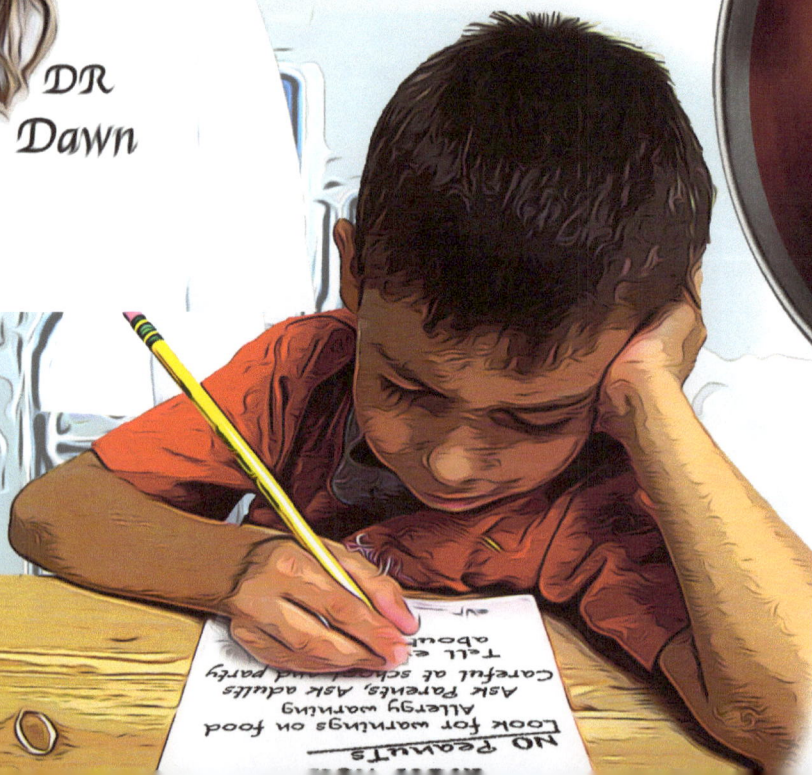

Look for warnings on food Allergy warning Ask Parents, Ask adults Careful at school and party Tell e about

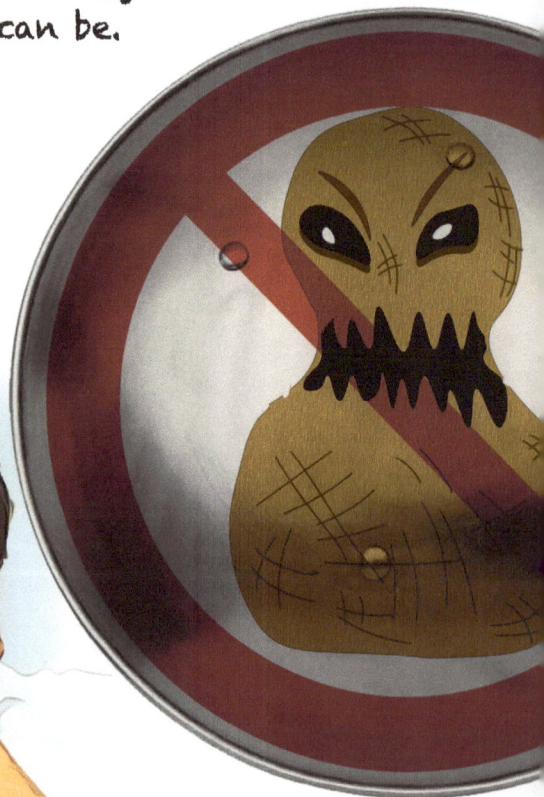

Elliot wrote everything the doctor said on a piece of paper

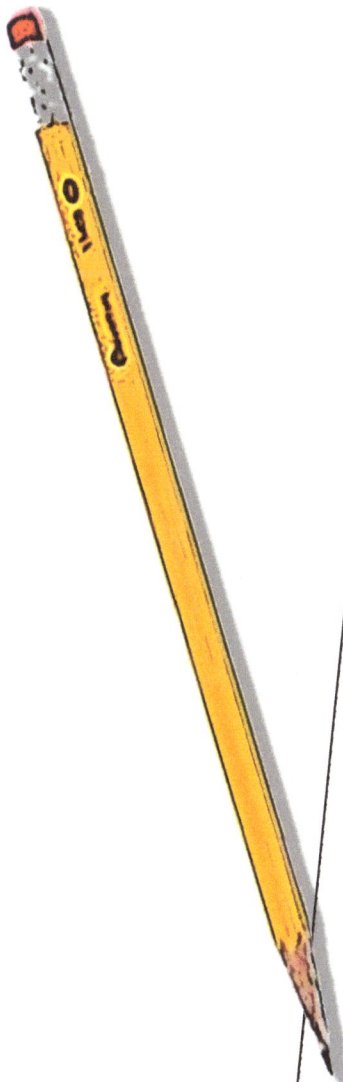

Elliot's allergies:
AVOID NUTS!
No Peanuts.

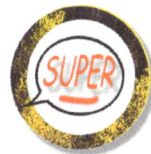

- Look for food allergy warnings, ask parents, ask adults.
  - Be careful at school and parties. **Tell everyone about the allergy.**

Check for signs of allergies:
Tingling or itching in the mouth; itchy, red, bumpy skin; swelling of the lips, face, tongue, and throat; wheezing, nasal congestion, or trouble breathing, abdominal pain, diarrhea, nausea or vomiting, and dizziness.

ALWAYS CARRY EPINEPHRINE PEN

SUPER

Stay Safe

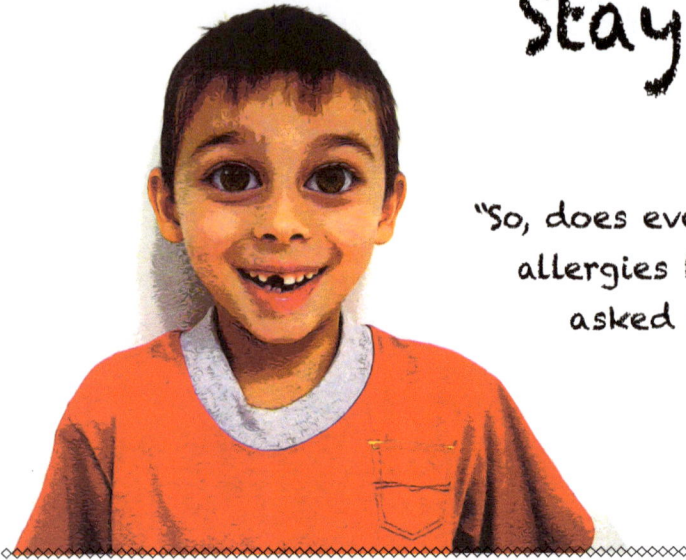

"So, does everyone have allergies like me?" asked Elliot.

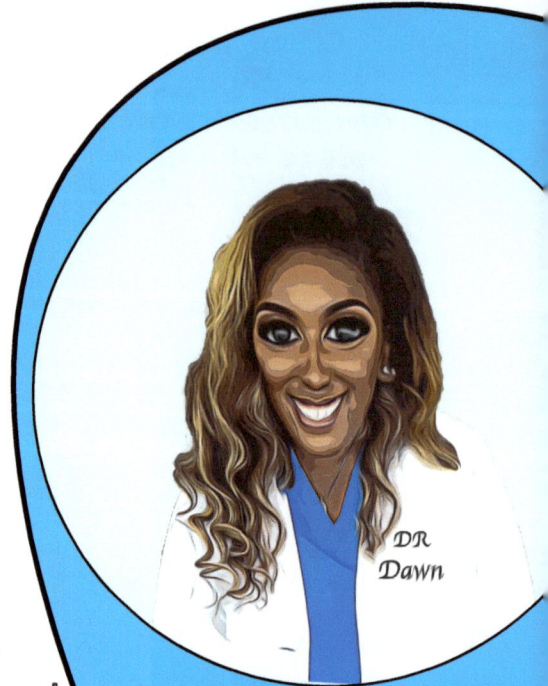

"Not everyone! About one in thirteen kids have a food allergy and each person is different with how they react to their allergy. You had a very bad reaction causing you to have a hard time breathing and your eyes got red and puffy. That is why you will need a special device called an epinephrine auto-injector(pen), similar to the pinch you got in the ambulance.

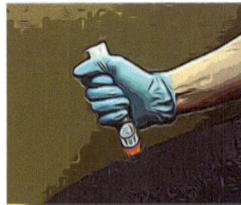

Many brands exist and should be discussed with your doctor"

DR Dawn

Take Control

The doctor talked to the whole family about how to be more aware of what they put in their body, and the importance of reading labels. It's not just about keeping away from foods with nuts, but also avoiding foods that come into contact with nuts in the factory where they are made.

The doctor gave Elliot a sticker and told him to remember that he is just like Superman and has to be very careful with what he eats.

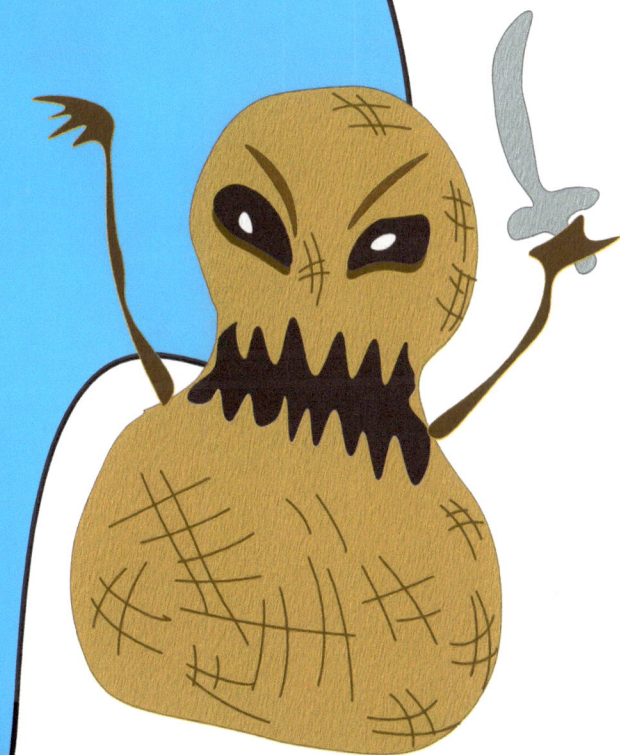

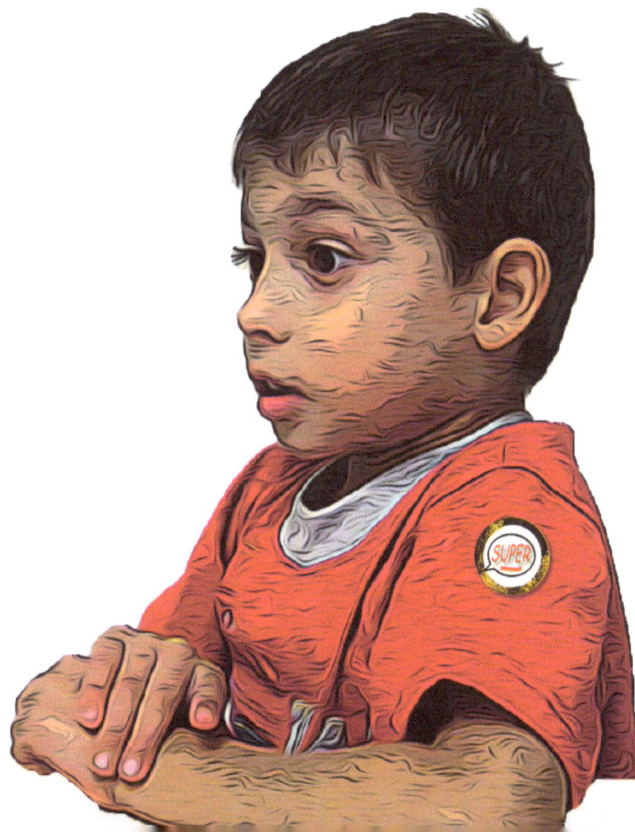

21

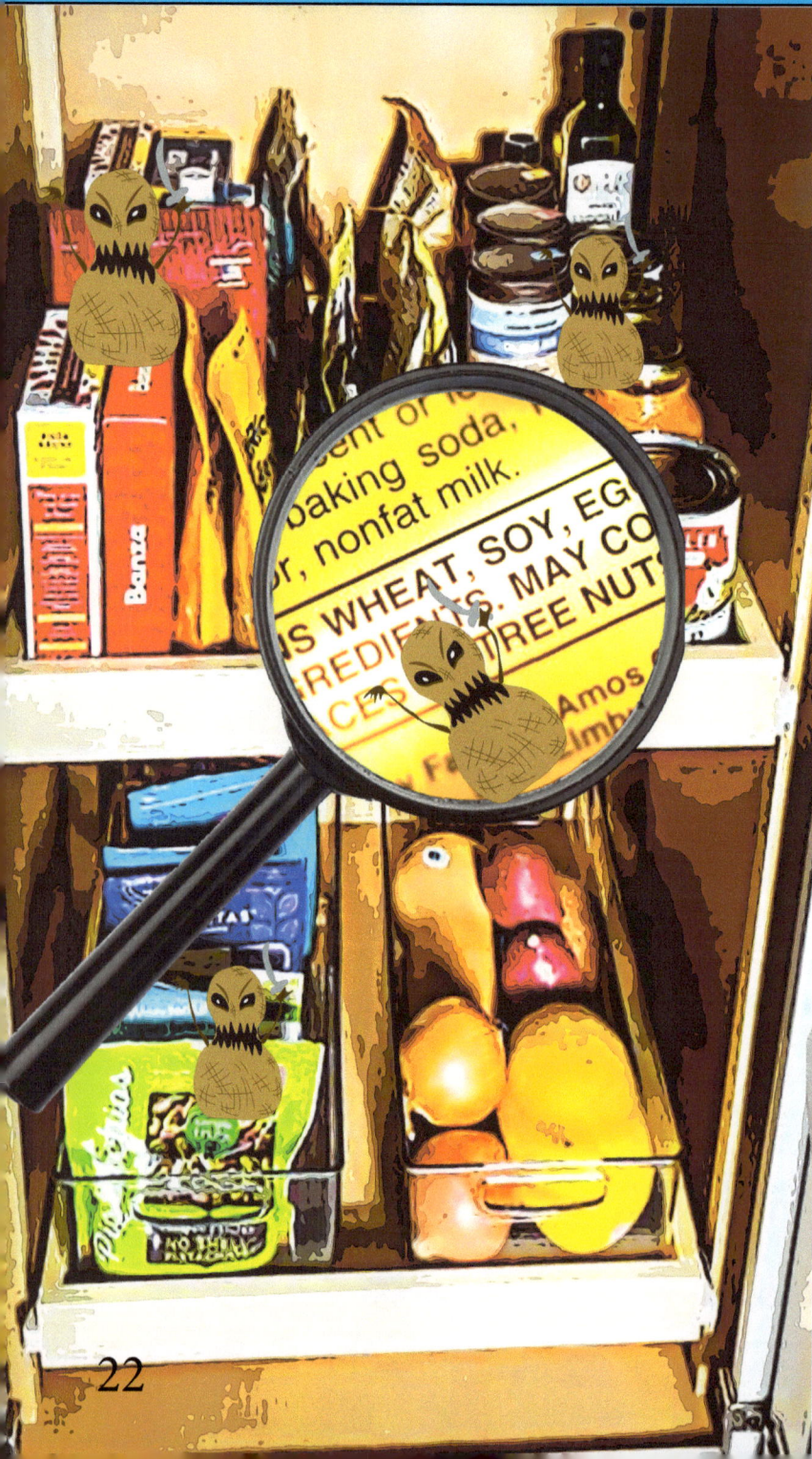

The Hunt

When the family returned home everyone started looking through the kitchen shelves and pantry to identify foods that either contained nuts or were made in a facility that also makes food with nuts.

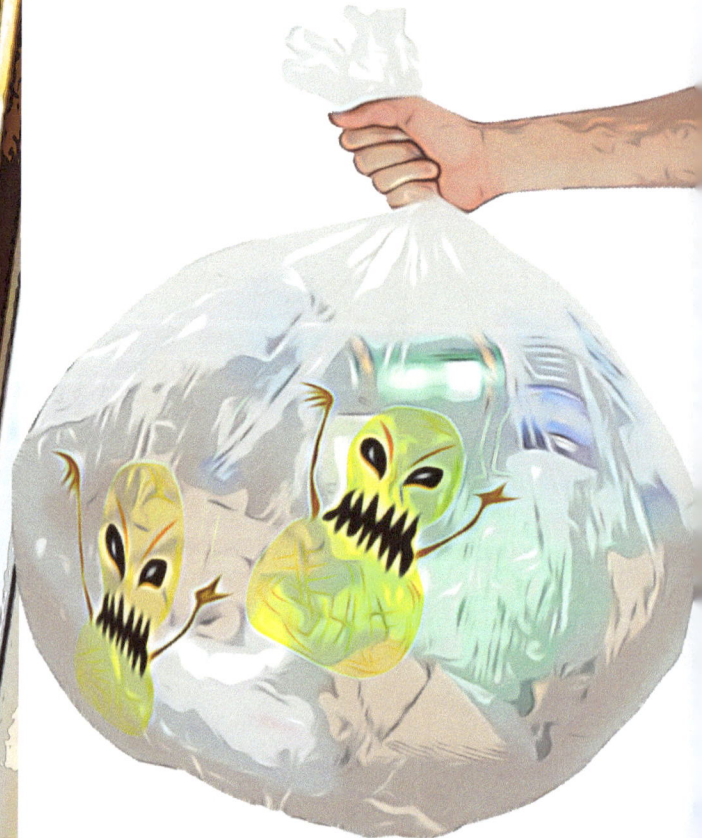

Sweet Dreams

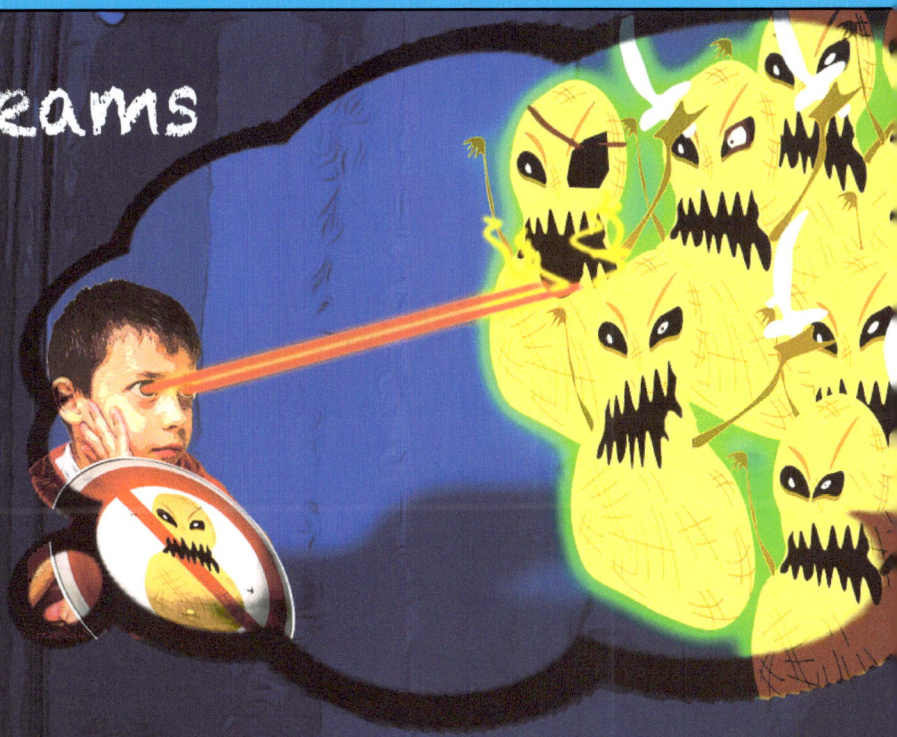

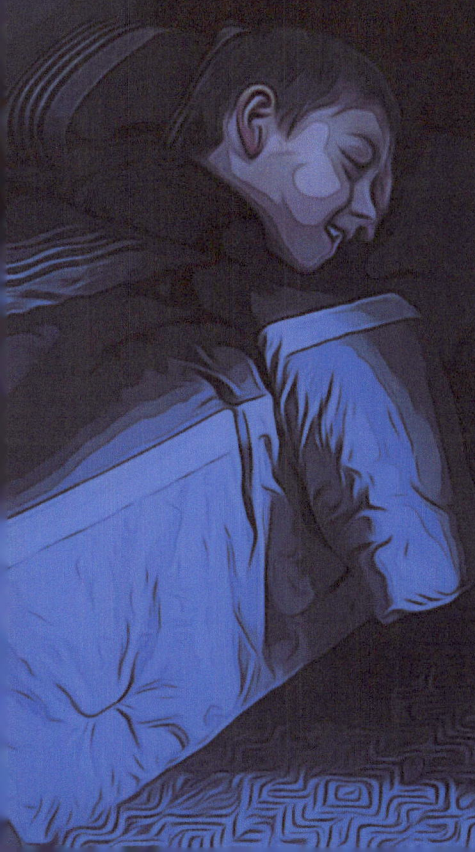

Elliot was very tired from all the excitement today.
When he went to bed, Mama kissed and hugged him
very tight and said,
"You were very brave today, my little Peanut."
"Mama, I don't want to be called Peanut anymore,"
Elliot said.
Mama smiled and said, "Okay my little superhero!"

Elliot went to bed dreaming of adventures
that he would have as a superhero.

Elliot's Tips

ALWAYS CARRY YOUR EPINEPHRINE PEN

Epinephrine is the only treatment that will stop a severe allergic reaction known as anaphylaxis [AN·A·PHY·LAX·IS].

Epinephrine comes as an auto-injector or a syringe and is manufactured by many differnt companies. It is only available through a prescription from your doctor.

BE AWARE AND HELP OTHERS

Many severe allergic reactions happen at schools and to children that were not diagnosed with allergies.

It is important to be aware of the signs and notify an adult immedietly to call 911 if you see someone with red bumpy skin, swelling of the lips, face or throat; wheezing or trouble breathing.

24

- Read before you eat!
- Always read labels for allergy information
- Even if you are familiar with the product, always read the label

Nutrition Facts

Serving Size 1 Bar (22g)

Amount Per Serving

Calories 90   Calories from Fat 20

	%Daily Value*
Total Fat 2g	3%
Saturated Fat 0g	0%
Trans Fat 0g	
Cholesterol 0mg	0%
Sodium 100mg	0%
Total Carbohydrate 16g	4%
Dietary Fiber 3g	10%
Sugars 6g	
Protein Ig	

Vitamin A	0%	Vitamin C	0%
Calcium	0%	Iron	0%
Thiamin	10%	Riboflavin	10%
Niacin	10%	Vitamin B6	10%

*Percent Dat values are based on a 2,000 calorie diet. Your daily values may be Higher or lower dependng on your calorie needs,

	Calories	2,000	2,500
Total Fat	Less than	65g	80g
Saturated Fat	Less than	20g	25g
Cholesterol	Less than	300mg	300mg
Sodium	Less than	2,400mg	2,400mg
Total Carbohydrate		300g	375g
Dietary Fiber		25g	30g

INGREDIENTS: CEREAL RICE, WHOLE GRAIN WHEAT, SUGAR, WHEAT BRAN. SOLUBLE WHEAT FIBER, SALT, MALT FLAVORING, VITAMIN BI [THIAMN MONONITRATE], VITAMIN B2,[RIBO-FLAVIN], SOLUBLE CORN FIBER, FRUCTOSE CORN SYRUP, ROASTED ALMONDS, ROASTED PEANUTS(PEANUTS,PEANUT OIL), SUNFLOWER OIL, DEXTROSE, SUGAR, HONEY CONTAINS 2% OR LESS OF SORBITOL, GLYCERIN, NATURAL AND ARTIFICIAL FLAVOR, SALT, SOY LECITHIN NIACINAMIDE, BHT (PRESERVATIVE), SOY PROTEIN ISOLATE, NONFAT MILK, VITAMIN Be (PYRIDOXINE HYDROCHLORIDE).

ALLERGY INFORMATION: CONTAINS WHEAT ALMOND, PEANUT, SOY AND MILK. MAY CONTAIN OTHER TREE-NUTS.

1

HOW TO READ THE INGREDIENTS?

1

Go to the bottom of the label, after the ingredients list, and look for a section called "Allergy Information." This will list common items that are considered allergens for people. Also, scan for phrases like "made on shared equipment" or "processed in the same facility".

Depending on how severe your allergy is, you may need to avoid the product. Manufacturers are frequently changing where and how they manufacture food, so always read the label like it is the first time you are reading it. After a few times, you will become really good at identifying allergens.